# Navigating Alzheimer's Future

## From Genomic Breakthroughs to Holistic Hope - A Comprehensive Guide

### By

### Fletcher Paul

# Table of contents

# Introduction

Alzheimer's disease, a formidable foe within the realm of neurodegenerative disorders, has captivated the attention of scientists, healthcare professionals, and society at large. This chapter serves as the gateway into the intricate world of Alzheimer's, aiming to unravel the mysteries that shroud this condition. Through an exploration of its history, biological underpinnings, and societal impact, we embark on a journey that seeks to demystify Alzheimer's disease.

# Understanding Alzheimer's Disease

At the heart of comprehending Alzheimer's lies an exploration of its fundamental nature. The disease, first identified by Dr. Alois Alzheimer in the early 20th century, manifests primarily as a progressive deterioration of cognitive function. The hallmark characteristics include memory loss, impaired judgment, and a decline in reasoning abilities. As we delve into the intricate web of neural changes, understanding the structural and chemical alterations in the brain becomes paramount.

Alzheimer's is intricately linked to the accumulation of abnormal protein deposits, specifically beta-amyloid plaques and tau tangles. These pathological entities disrupt normal neuronal communication and trigger a cascade of events leading to cognitive decline. The unraveling of these processes is crucial for developing targeted interventions and advancing our comprehension of the disease trajectory.

Beyond the biological aspects, understanding the human experience of Alzheimer's is equally imperative.By merging scientific insights with lived experiences, a holistic understanding of

Alzheimer's disease emerges, fostering empathy and a nuanced perspective.

## Significance of Research

The significance of Alzheimer's research reverberates through both scientific and societal spheres. With an aging global population, the prevalence of Alzheimer's is escalating, presenting an urgent need for effective interventions. Research endeavors are multifaceted, encompassing a quest for early detection methods, innovative treatment modalities, and a deeper understanding of the disease's heterogeneity.

In the quest for a cure, the significance of genetic and environmental factors cannot be overstated. This subsection delves into the genetic predispositions that elevate the risk of Alzheimer's, providing insights into familial patterns and hereditary influences. Concurrently, it scrutinizes the environmental factors—ranging from lifestyle choices to exposure to toxins—that contribute to the disease's onset and progression.

The societal impact of Alzheimer's underscores the critical importance of research. As the disease places an increasing burden on healthcare systems and caregivers, understanding its economic and social ramifications becomes pivotal. The significance of research extends beyond the laboratory, encompassing advocacy, public awareness, and destigmatization efforts. By elucidating the societal implications of Alzheimer's, this chapter aims to underscore the imperative nature of continued research, weaving a narrative that intertwines scientific pursuit with the betterment of individuals and communities affected by the disease.

# Chapter 2: Historical Overview

Alzheimer's disease has a rich and intricate history that intertwines scientific discovery, medical breakthroughs, and the evolving understanding of cognitive disorders. This chapter delves into the annals of time to explore the historical journey of Alzheimer's, from its discovery to key milestones in research.

## Discovery and Early Observations

The genesis of Alzheimer's disease traces back to the early 20th century when Dr. Alois Alzheimer, a German psychiatrist and neuropathologist, made a groundbreaking observation. In 1906, Dr. Alzheimer presented a case study involving a middle-aged woman named Auguste Deter, whose cognitive decline was marked by memory loss, language difficulties, and erratic behavior. Upon her death, an autopsy revealed distinctive abnormalities in her brain, laying the foundation for the identification of a novel neurological disorder.

This section delves into the meticulous documentation of Auguste Deter's case and Dr. Alzheimer's subsequent research. It explores the initial challenges faced in comprehending this enigmatic condition, emphasizing the significance of these early observations in shaping the understanding of Alzheimer's disease.

## Milestones in Alzheimer's Research

The journey from the initial discovery to contemporary research is marked by numerous milestones that have significantly advanced our comprehension of Alzheimer's. This subsection chronicles key breakthroughs, highlighting pivotal moments that have reshaped the landscape of Alzheimer's research.

One such milestone is the identification of beta-amyloid plaques and tau tangles—the pathological hallmarks of Alzheimer's—in the 1980s. This discovery ushered in a new era of understanding, paving the way for targeted therapeutic approaches. The elucidation of the genetic component, particularly the APOE gene's role, furthered our understanding of the disease's hereditary aspects.

Advancements in neuroimaging techniques, such as PET and MRI scans, have allowed researchers to visualize and track the progression of Alzheimer's in living brains. Additionally, the establishment of large-scale collaborative initiatives, like the Alzheimer's Disease Neuroimaging Initiative (ADNI), has facilitated data sharing and accelerated research efforts.

As we traverse through these milestones, it becomes evident that Alzheimer's research is a dynamic and collaborative endeavor, with each breakthrough building upon the knowledge gained from preceding achievements. This section aims to provide a comprehensive narrative that underscores the significance of historical milestones in shaping our current understanding of Alzheimer's disease.

# Chapter 3: The Biology of Alzheimer's

Alzheimer's disease is fundamentally a disorder of the brain, characterized by intricate changes in its structure and function. This chapter delves into the biological underpinnings of Alzheimer's, exploring the complexities of brain anatomy, the normal functions it serves, and the specific neurological alterations that define this progressive disorder.

# Brain Structure and Function

Understanding the biology of Alzheimer's necessitates a journey into the intricacies of brain structure and function. The brain, the epicenter of cognitive abilities, is a marvel of complexity. This section elucidates the various regions of the brain responsible for memory, cognition, and emotional processing. A particular focus is placed on the hippocampus, amygdala, and neocortex, as these regions play pivotal roles in the manifestations of Alzheimer's disease.

By unraveling the normal functioning of these brain regions, we lay the groundwork for comprehending the devastating impact Alzheimer's has on cognitive processes. The intricate network of neurons, synapses, and neurotransmitters forms the tapestry of cognitive function, and deviations from this delicate balance become apparent in the progression of Alzheimer's.

## Neurological Changes in Alzheimer's

At the heart of Alzheimer's pathology lie the distinctive neurological changes that distinguish it from normal brain aging. This section scrutinizes the abnormal protein accumulations—beta-amyloid plaques and tau tangles—that infiltrate the brain, disrupting neuronal communication and integrity.

Beta-amyloid, typically involved in synaptic function, misfolds and aggregates, forming plaques that interfere with normal cellular processes. Simultaneously, tau, a microtubule-stabilizing protein, undergoes abnormal phosphorylation, leading to the formation of tangles that contribute to neuronal degeneration. The interconnected nature of these pathological changes sets the stage for cognitive decline and the characteristic symptoms of Alzheimer's.

As we navigate through the neurological intricacies of Alzheimer's, this chapter strives to bridge the gap between the microscopic abnormalities and the macroscopic impact on cognitive abilities. By comprehending the biological nuances, we pave the way for targeted therapeutic interventions and a deeper appreciation of the challenges posed by Alzheimer's disease.

# Chapter 4: Causes and Risk Factors

Alzheimer's disease, a complex and multifaceted neurodegenerative condition, is influenced by an intricate interplay of genetic, environmental, and lifestyle factors. Understanding the causes and risk factors associated with Alzheimer's is crucial for both preventative efforts and the development of targeted interventions. This chapter embarks on an exploration of the diverse elements that contribute to the onset and progression of Alzheimer's, unraveling the genetic predispositions, environmental impacts, and lifestyle choices that shape its complex landscape.

## Genetic Factors

Genetic factors are key determinants in the susceptibility to Alzheimer's disease, providing a unique window into understanding familial patterns and hereditary influences. The APOE gene, identified as a significant genetic risk factor, is explored in depth. Individuals carrying certain variations of this gene face an increased risk of developing Alzheimer's, shedding light on the intricate genetic landscape.

The chapter delves into the historical context of genetic research on Alzheimer's, from the initial identification of APOE as a risk gene to the ongoing exploration of other genetic markers. Researchers are uncovering additional genes associated with Alzheimer's, contributing to a more nuanced understanding of the intricate genetic web that underlies the disease.

The emerging field of genetic research holds promise for personalized medicine and targeted interventions. By understanding an individual's genetic makeup, healthcare providers can potentially tailor treatments to address specific genetic vulnerabilities. This section emphasizes the importance of ongoing genetic research in refining our understanding of Alzheimer's and paving the way for more precise and effective therapeutic strategies.

## Environmental Influences

Beyond genetics, environmental influences exert a significant impact on Alzheimer's risk. This section navigates through the various external factors that contribute to the complex tapestry of Alzheimer's susceptibility. From exposure to pollutants to the impact of educational opportunities, the environment plays a crucial role in shaping an individual's risk profile.

The exploration extends to the role of cognitive stimulation and social engagement as protective environmental factors. Studies suggest that an intellectually stimulating environment and strong social connections may contribute to cognitive resilience and delay the onset of Alzheimer's symptoms. This highlights the importance of a holistic approach to understanding the environmental influences that impact cognitive health.

The section underscores the modifiable nature of some environmental factors. By identifying and addressing these factors, there may be opportunities for prevention and intervention. The discussion encompasses the impact of lifestyle choices, access to education, and socio-economic factors, providing a comprehensive overview of the environmental components that contribute to Alzheimer's risk.

## Lifestyle and Alzheimer's

Lifestyle choices, encompassing diet, physical activity, and cognitive engagement, form a crucial dimension of

Alzheimer's risk. This section delves into the intricate connections between lifestyle factors and cognitive health, exploring how individual choices may influence susceptibility to the disease.

Dietary patterns, such as the Mediterranean diet, have been associated with a lower risk of Alzheimer's. The role of antioxidants, omega-3 fatty acids, and other nutritional elements in promoting brain health is explored. Additionally, the impact of physical exercise on cognitive function is discussed, highlighting the potential benefits of an active lifestyle in mitigating Alzheimer's risk.

Cognitive engagement, including activities that stimulate the brain, is presented as a proactive measure against Alzheimer's. Mental exercises, lifelong learning, and engaging in intellectually stimulating pursuits may contribute to cognitive reserve, providing a buffer against the pathological changes associated with the disease.

By scrutinizing the intricate connections between lifestyle choices and Alzheimer's risk, this section aims to empower individuals with the knowledge to make informed decisions. The discussion not only underscores the risks associated with sedentary behavior and poor dietary choices but also emphasizes the potential for lifestyle modifications as a means of promoting brain health and potentially reducing the risk of Alzheimer's.

In conclusion, this chapter provides a comprehensive exploration of the causes and risk factors associated with Alzheimer's disease. By unraveling the genetic, environmental, and lifestyle elements that contribute to its complexity, we gain valuable insights into the diverse factors shaping the landscape of Alzheimer's susceptibility. This understanding is instrumental in guiding both preventative measures and future research efforts aimed at developing targeted interventions for this challenging and prevalent neurodegenerative disorder.

# Chapter 5: Diagnosis and Early Detection

Alzheimer's disease, a progressive neurodegenerative disorder, poses a significant challenge for early detection due to its insidious onset. Timely diagnosis is crucial for implementing interventions that can slow its progression and enhance the quality of life for affected individuals. This chapter delves into the complex landscape of diagnosing Alzheimer's, exploring the methodologies, tools, and advancements in cognitive assessment, medical imaging, and biomarkers that contribute to the early detection of this challenging condition.

## Cognitive Assessment

The diagnosis of Alzheimer's often begins with a comprehensive cognitive assessment, a process that involves evaluating an individual's cognitive abilities and detecting any deviations from the normal range. These assessments serve as vital tools in identifying the subtle cognitive changes indicative of Alzheimer's disease.

Cognitive tests, such as the Mini-Mental State Examination (MMSE) and the

Montreal Cognitive Assessment (MoCA), play a central role in this process. The MMSE assesses various cognitive domains, including orientation, memory, attention, language, and visuospatial abilities. Similarly, the MoCA, a more sensitive tool, delves deeper into executive function and higher-level cognitive tasks.

However, conducting cognitive assessments is not without challenges. Factors such as cultural diversity, educational background, and linguistic differences can influence test performance. This section of the chapter delves into the nuances of cognitive assessment, highlighting the importance of considering these factors in the diagnostic process. It also explores the ongoing efforts to develop and validate culturally sensitive and educationally unbiased cognitive assessments, aiming to improve the accuracy and inclusivity of Alzheimer's diagnosis.

Additionally, this section discusses the role of emerging technologies, such as digital cognitive assessments and virtual reality-based tests, in enhancing the sensitivity and specificity of early cognitive screening. The incorporation of these innovative approaches holds promise for more accurate and personalized assessments, addressing some of the limitations associated with traditional cognitive tests.

## Imaging and Biomarkers

Advancements in medical imaging have transformed our ability to visualize and understand the structural and functional changes in the brain associated with Alzheimer's disease. This section of the chapter explores the use of imaging techniques, including Magnetic Resonance Imaging (MRI) and Positron Emission Tomography (PET), in the diagnostic process.

MRI provides detailed images of the brain's structure, helping clinicians rule out other potential causes of cognitive decline and identify specific abnormalities associated with Alzheimer's. PET scans, utilizing radiotracers that bind to beta-amyloid plaques and tau tangles, offer a means of visualizing these pathological hallmarks in living brains, contributing to a more accurate diagnosis.

The discussion extends to the evolving landscape of biomarkers, measurable indicators that reflect biological processes associated with Alzheimer's disease. Cerebrospinal fluid (CSF) biomarkers, such as beta-amyloid and tau proteins, provide valuable insights into the molecular changes occurring in the brain. Blood-based biomarkers are emerging as promising alternatives, offering a less invasive and more accessible option for early detection.

Despite the potential of biomarkers, challenges persist in standardizing their use and addressing issues related to accessibility and cost. Ongoing research endeavors focus on refining and validating biomarker panels to enhance their reliability in predicting Alzheimer's risk and progression.

The chapter underscores the significance of combining cognitive assessments with imaging and biomarkers for a comprehensive diagnostic approach. Integrating multiple modalities increases the accuracy and reliability of early detection, allowing for a more nuanced understanding of Alzheimer's disease.

In conclusion, this chapter provides an in-depth exploration of the diagnostic landscape for Alzheimer's disease, with a specific focus on cognitive assessment, medical imaging, and biomarkers. The evolving methodologies and advancements discussed underscore the ongoing commitment to improving early detection strategies. As research continues to unravel the complexities of Alzheimer's, the integration of these diagnostic tools holds promise for a future where early intervention becomes a reality, offering hope for improved outcomes and a better quality of life for those affected by this challenging neurological disorder.

# Chapter 6: Stages of Alzheimer's

Alzheimer's disease unfolds progressively through discernible stages, each characterized by unique patterns of cognitive decline and functional impairment. This chapter delves into the nuanced progression of Alzheimer's, traversing from mild cognitive impairment through the early, middle, and late stages. Grasping this trajectory is essential for caregivers, healthcare professionals, and individuals affected by Alzheimer's, offering insights into the evolving nature of the disease and guiding appropriate support and care.

## Mild Cognitive Impairment

Initiating the Alzheimer's journey, Mild Cognitive Impairment (MCI) signifies the early stage marked by subtle cognitive changes exceeding typical age-related decline but not significantly impacting daily functioning. This section explores the delicate equilibrium between normal aging and the initial signs of Alzheimer's, underscoring the importance of recognizing MCI as a potential precursor to more severe cognitive decline.

MCI manifests with memory lapses, challenges in decision-making, and concentration difficulties. However, these changes are subtle and may not significantly disrupt daily activities. This portion delves into MCI diagnostic criteria, the complexities of differentiating it from age-related cognitive changes, and ongoing research refining our comprehension of this transitional stage.

Furthermore, the chapter addresses the variability in MCI progression to Alzheimer's, acknowledging not everyone with MCI advances to a more severe stage. Some individuals remain stable, while others may revert to normal cognitive functioning. This uncertainty underscores the need for continual monitoring and personalized care plans tailored to individuals experiencing MCI.

## Early, Middle, and Late Stages

The trajectory of Alzheimer's unfolds through distinct stages, each marked by specific cognitive, functional, and behavioral changes. This segment navigates through the early, middle, and late stages, offering a comprehensive overview of the disease's evolving nature.

**Early Stage:** Characterized by noticeable cognitive decline, individuals encounter challenges in memory, language, and problem-solving. This part explores the hurdles faced by those in the early stage, grappling with awareness of cognitive changes. It also emphasizes the significance of early diagnosis, enabling active participation in care planning and decision-making.

**Middle Stage:** As Alzheimer's progresses to the middle stage, cognitive decline intensifies, impacting daily activities and independence. This section delves into the challenges for both individuals and caregivers during the middle stage, managing changes in behavior, communication difficulties, and the growing need for assistance with daily tasks. Strategies for providing supportive care and maintaining quality of life are discussed.

**Late Stage:** Representing the most advanced phase, the late stage is debilitating, with individuals requiring extensive assistance for daily activities, losing verbal communication, and experiencing a significant decline in physical functioning. This portion explores the profound impact on individuals and caregivers during the late stage, emphasizing the importance of compassionate and person-centered care.

Throughout these stages, the chapter underscores the variability in individual experiences, acknowledging that Alzheimer's progression is distinctive for each person. It also discusses the emotional and practical challenges faced by caregivers, highlighting the importance of a holistic and personalized approach to care.

Concluding, this chapter provides a detailed exploration of Alzheimer's stages, from mild cognitive impairment through the early, middle, and late stages. Understanding the distinct characteristics and challenges at each stage enables caregivers, healthcare professionals, and individuals affected by Alzheimer's to navigate the complexities of the disease with greater insight and empathy. This knowledge forms the basis for tailored care plans, support systems, and advocacy efforts to enhance the lives of those impacted by Alzheimer's throughout its progressive stages.

# Chapter 7: Treatment Approaches

Alzheimer's complaint presently lacks a cure, and available treatments offer fairly modest characteristic benefits, primarily of a palliative nature. This chapter explores the different treatment approaches for Alzheimer's, dividing them into medicine and non-pharmacological interventions, furnishing a comprehensive overview of the strategies employed to address the complications of this grueling condition.

# Medications

## Acetylcholinesterase Impediments and Memantine

Medicine play a vital part in managing the cognitive symptoms of Alzheimer's complaint. Acetylcholinesterase impediments, including tacrine, rivastigmine, galantamine, and donepezil, are designed to treat mild to severe Alzheimer's. These medicines aim to offset the reduction in cholinergic neuron exertion, a notable point of Alzheimer's, by decelerating down the breakdown of acetylcholine( ACh). still, the benefits deduced from their use are fairly small, and common side goods include nausea and vomiting, linked to cholinergic excess. Another class of drug, memantine, acts as an NMDA receptor antagonist, addressing the part of glutamate in Alzheimer's pathology. By blocking NMDA receptors and precluding excitotoxicity, memantine has shown a small benefit in treating moderate to severe Alzheimer's complaint. Adverse events with memantine are occasional and mild, similar as visions, confusion, dizziness, headache, and fatigue. The combination of memantine and donepezil has demonstrated statistically significant but clinically borderline effectiveness.

## Ginkgo Biloba Extract( EGb 761) and Atypical Antipsychotics

Ginkgo biloba excerpt, known as EGb 761, has been employed in treating Alzheimer's and other neuropsychiatric diseases. Approved throughout Europe, EGb 761 has shown enhancement in symptoms for both Alzheimer's complaint and vascular madness. still, a 2016 review indicated inadequate substantiation from clinical trials to warrant its use medicinally for Alzheimer's complaint. Atypical antipsychotics, while modestly useful in reducing aggression and psychosis in individualities with Alzheimer's, come with serious adverse goods, including stroke, movement difficulties, and cognitive decline. Dragged use has been associated with increased mortality. termination of antipsychotic use appears to be safe in this population.

## Non-Pharmacological Interventions

**Psychosocial Interventions** Non-pharmacological interventions play a pivotal part as adjuncts to pharmaceutical treatment. Psychosocial interventions encompass behaviour -, emotion-, cognition-, or stimulation-acquainted approaches. Behavioral interventions concentrate on relating and reducing antecedents and consequences of problem actions, offering targeted support for specific challenges, similar as incontinence. Emotion- acquainted interventions include reminiscence remedy, confirmation remedy, probative psychotherapy, sensitive integration( snoezelen), and dissembled presence remedy. Reminiscence remedy involves agitating once gests , frequently with the aid of familiar particulars. Simulated presence remedy uses recordings of close cousins' voices to reduce grueling actions. Cognition- acquainted treatments, similar as reality exposure and cognitive retraining, aim to reduce cognitive poverties. Reality exposure provides information about time, place, or person to enhance understanding of surroundings. Cognitive retraining exercises internal capacities, showing some efficacity in perfecting cognitive capacities. Stimulation- acquainted treatments, including art, music, and pet curatives, exercise, and recreational conditioning, offer modest support for perfecting behaviour, mood, and function. The main benefit lies in the change to the person's routine, contributing to overall well- being. In conclusion, this chapter delves into the different treatment approaches for

Alzheimer's complaint, encompassing both pharmaceutical interventions and non-pharmacological strategies. While medicine target cognitive symptoms,non-pharmacological interventions play a vital part in enhancing overall well-being, addressing specific challenges, and furnishing a holistic approach to watch for individualities and their caregivers affected by Alzheimer's.

# Chapter 8: Caregiving Challenges

Caring for individuals with Alzheimer's disease is a profound and demanding responsibility that extends beyond the realms of physical care. This chapter explores the intricate challenges faced by caregivers, encompassing both emotional and practical aspects of caregiving, while emphasizing the pivotal role of robust support systems in navigating this complex journey.

# Emotional and Practical Aspects

## Emotional Challenges in Caregiving

Caring for a loved one with Alzheimer's disease presents a unique set of emotional challenges that caregivers must navigate. Witnessing the cognitive decline of someone close can evoke a range of emotions, from grief and frustration to anxiety and stress. The emotional toll is particularly poignant as caregivers grapple with the gradual loss of the person they once knew.

Grief becomes a constant companion as caregivers mourn the diminishing abilities and changing personality of the individual with Alzheimer's. This section delves into the emotional landscape of caregiving, highlighting the importance of acknowledging and processing these complex emotions. Caregivers often find solace in support groups or individual counseling, providing a safe space to express their feelings and connect with others who share similar experiences.

Frustration is a common sentiment as caregivers face the daily challenges of communication breakdowns, repetitive behaviors, and the unpredictability of Alzheimer's symptoms. Understanding the nature of the disease and learning effective coping strategies becomes essential for emotional resilience. The chapter explores various approaches, such as mindfulness techniques and stress-management practices, to help caregivers navigate the emotional highs and lows.

## Practical Challenges in Caregiving

The practical aspects of caregiving are equally demanding, requiring caregivers to adapt to the evolving needs of individuals with Alzheimer's. Daily tasks that were once routine can become intricate challenges, necessitating modifications to the living environment and lifestyle.

Simplifying routines and creating a structured daily schedule are practical adjustments that enhance the quality of life for both the caregiver and the person with Alzheimer's. Safety measures, such as using safety locks and labeling household items, contribute to a secure living environment. This section explores the importance of adapting the physical space to align with the cognitive abilities of the individual, promoting independence while ensuring safety.

Meal preparation becomes a significant practical challenge, especially as eating habits change. The need for smaller, more manageable pieces of food or pureed options may arise. The chapter discusses practical strategies for addressing dietary challenges and ensuring proper nutrition.

Swallowing difficulties can further complicate the practical aspects of caregiving, potentially requiring the use of feeding tubes. Caregivers and family members must grapple with the medical efficacy and ethical considerations of continuing feeding interventions. This section navigates the delicate balance between ensuring the well-being of the individual and making ethically sound decisions.

## Support for Caregivers

## Formal Support Systems

Recognizing the multifaceted demands of caregiving, this section underscores the crucial need for support systems to alleviate the challenges faced by caregivers. Formal support structures, such as respite care, provide caregivers with temporary relief, allowing them to rejuvenate and prevent burnout. The chapter explores the importance of accessing these formal support services and the positive impact they have on both caregivers and those they care for.

## Informal Support and Communication

Informal support from family and friends is invaluable in the caregiving journey. Open communication within the caregiver's network fosters understanding and collaboration, creating a cohesive support system. This section emphasizes the significance of sharing responsibilities and ensuring that caregivers feel supported and connected within their social circles.

Community resources, including Alzheimer's associations and local support groups, play a vital role in providing guidance and a sense of community for caregivers. The chapter explores the wealth of information and support available through these channels, highlighting their importance in creating a network of shared experiences and practical advice.

## Self-Care for Caregivers

As caregiving can be all-encompassing, this section emphasizes the crucial aspect of self-care for caregivers. Balancing the responsibilities of caregiving with personal well-being is essential for maintaining overall health. Strategies for self-care, ranging from taking breaks and maintaining hobbies to prioritizing mental and physical health, are explored in-depth. This chapter reinforces the notion that caregivers must prioritize their own well-being to provide effective and sustainable care to their loved ones.

In conclusion, this chapter provides a comprehensive exploration of the emotional and practical challenges inherent in caregiving for individuals with Alzheimer's disease. By delving into the nuanced aspects of caregiving, it seeks to equip caregivers with insights and strategies to navigate the complexities of their role. The section on support underscores the need for a collaborative approach, recognizing that caregivers are not alone in their journey and that a robust support system is essential for fostering resilience and enhancing the well-being of both caregivers and those they care for.

# Chapter 9: Research Advances

Research into Alzheimer's disease is at the forefront of scientific inquiry, driven by the urgent need to unravel its complexities, discover effective treatments, and ultimately find a cure. This chapter explores the latest advancements in Alzheimer's research, delving into current studies and findings while highlighting promising areas of research that offer hope for the future.

# Current Studies and Findings

## Unraveling the Genetic Tapestry

Current studies in Alzheimer's research are making significant strides in understanding the genetic underpinnings of the disease. Researchers are delving into the intricate genetic tapestry that contributes to Alzheimer's risk and progression. Large-scale genomic studies, such as genome-wide association studies (GWAS), have identified specific genetic variants associated with an increased susceptibility to Alzheimer's. These findings provide crucial insights into the biological mechanisms underlying the disease.

Furthermore, the exploration of genetic mutations linked to familial Alzheimer's disease is shedding light on the intricate interplay between genetic factors and the onset of the condition. Advances in gene-editing technologies, such as CRISPR-Cas9, are opening new avenues for manipulating specific genes associated with Alzheimer's in experimental settings. These technologies hold promise for targeted interventions and personalized treatments in the future.

## Biomarkers for Early Detection

Early detection of Alzheimer's disease is a key focus of current research efforts. Biomarkers—measurable indicators of biological processes—are emerging as valuable tools for identifying the disease in its early stages. Cerebrospinal fluid and blood biomarkers, along with advanced imaging techniques such as positron emission tomography (PET) and magnetic resonance imaging (MRI), are providing researchers with the means to detect pathological changes associated with Alzheimer's before the onset of noticeable symptoms.

Studies are investigating the accuracy and reliability of these biomarkers in predicting Alzheimer's risk and tracking disease progression. The goal is to develop reliable diagnostic tools that enable early intervention and treatment, potentially altering the course of the disease before irreversible damage occurs.

## Immunotherapy and Disease Modification

Immunotherapy is a groundbreaking area of research in Alzheimer's, aiming to harness the body's immune system to target and clear the abnormal proteins— beta-amyloid plaques and tau tangles— that characterize the disease. Recent clinical trials testing immunotherapeutic approaches have shown promise in reducing the accumulation of these pathological proteins in the brains of individuals with Alzheimer's.

Monoclonal antibodies, designed to selectively bind and remove beta-amyloid, are among the leading candidates in immunotherapy research. Some studies have demonstrated a reduction in beta-amyloid levels and a slowing of cognitive decline in participants treated with these antibodies. However, challenges such as treatment timing, dosage optimization, and potential side effects remain focal points for further investigation.

# Promising Areas of Research

## Precision Medicine Approaches

The quest for precision medicine in Alzheimer's research involves tailoring treatments to individuals based on their unique genetic makeup, lifestyle, and other personal factors. Advances in understanding the genetic variability among individuals with Alzheimer's are paving the way for more targeted and personalized therapeutic interventions.

Current research is exploring the concept of stratified medicine, where specific subgroups of individuals with Alzheimer's are identified based on their genetic profiles. This approach allows for the development of targeted treatments designed to address the specific mechanisms driving the disease in each subgroup. Precision medicine offers the potential to enhance treatment efficacy while minimizing adverse effects, representing a paradigm shift towards more individualized care.

## Neuroinflammation and Microglial Activation

Neuroinflammation, characterized by the activation of immune cells in the brain, is a burgeoning area of interest in Alzheimer's research. Microglia, the resident immune cells in the brain, play a pivotal role in modulating neuroinflammatory responses. Recent studies are elucidating the complex interactions between neuroinflammation, the accumulation of pathological proteins, and cognitive decline in Alzheimer's.

Targeting microglial activation as a therapeutic strategy is gaining momentum. Researchers are exploring drugs that can modulate microglial function, either dampening excessive inflammation or enhancing the clearance of abnormal proteins. Understanding the delicate balance between protective and harmful aspects of neuroinflammation is critical for developing interventions that mitigate disease progression.

## Cognitive Reserve and Lifestyle Interventions

Cognitive reserve, the brain's ability to maintain function despite damage, is an intriguing aspect of Alzheimer's research. Studies suggest that lifestyle factors, such as education, cognitive engagement, and social activities, contribute to cognitive reserve and may influence the risk and progression of Alzheimer's.

Research is delving into the mechanisms through which cognitive reserve exerts its protective effects. Cognitive stimulation, physical exercise, and social engagement are emerging as potential modifiable factors that can enhance cognitive reserve. Understanding the impact of lifestyle interventions on brain health is opening new avenues for developing preventive strategies and holistic approaches to Alzheimer's care.

In conclusion, this chapter provides a comprehensive overview of the latest research advances in Alzheimer's disease. Current studies are unraveling the genetic complexities, exploring biomarkers for early detection, and investigating immunotherapy for disease modification. Promising areas of research include precision medicine approaches, the role of neuroinflammation and microglial activation, and the impact of cognitive reserve and lifestyle interventions. As the scientific community continues to deepen its understanding of Alzheimer's, these advances offer hope for more effective treatments, early interventions, and ultimately, a transformative impact on the lives of individuals affected by this challenging condition.

# Chapter 10: Alzheimer's and Society

Alzheimer's disease, a complex and challenging condition, transcends its individual impact, sending profound ripples throughout society. This chapter delves into the intricate relationship between Alzheimer's and society, exploring the social impact of the disease and the transformative potential of public awareness and advocacy.

# Social Impact

## The Ripple Effect on Families and Caregivers

Alzheimer's disease, with its gradual erosion of cognitive abilities, exerts a significant social impact, particularly within the realm of families and caregiving circles. This section illuminates the transformative journey within families, where roles undergo evolution, and relationships navigate the challenges posed by Alzheimer's. As individuals step into the role of caregivers, the emotional, financial, and practical burdens extend beyond the affected individual to touch the very core of familial dynamics.

Caregivers often find themselves navigating a landscape marked by social isolation. The demands of Alzheimer's caregiving can make routine social interactions challenging, and this section emphasizes the urgent need for comprehensive community support systems. Understanding the unique social dynamics created by Alzheimer's and addressing the emotional toll on caregivers are essential steps toward creating a more compassionate and supportive societal framework.

## Workplace Impacts and Economic Considerations

Beyond the familial sphere, Alzheimer's leaves an indelible mark on the workplace and the broader economic landscape. This part of the chapter delves into the intricate impacts on the professional lives of individuals affected by Alzheimer's and their caregivers. Cognitive decline, a hallmark of the disease, can influence productivity and necessitate workplace accommodations. The discussion emphasizes the necessity for workplace policies that accommodate the unique challenges posed by Alzheimer's and the economic considerations that arise from the disease's pervasive effects.

Economically, Alzheimer's imposes a substantial burden, spanning direct medical expenses, long-term care costs, and productivity losses. This section explores the economic implications borne by society and scrutinizes potential strategies for mitigating these costs. The call for research, policy interventions, and support mechanisms aims to alleviate the economic strain and foster a societal environment that responds empathetically to the challenges posed by Alzheimer's.

# Public Awareness and Advocacy

## Shaping Public Perception and Breaking Stigmas

Public awareness emerges as a potent force in the quest to transform societal responses to Alzheimer's disease. This subsection investigates the prevailing state of public perception and confronts the stigmas that often shroud Alzheimer's. Dispelling myths and misconceptions becomes a cornerstone, with accurate information serving as a powerful tool to shape a more compassionate and informed society.

Advocacy efforts play a pivotal role in elevating Alzheimer's on the public agenda. The section explores successful advocacy campaigns that have contributed to increased funding, improved legislation, and enhanced support systems. By urging policymakers, healthcare professionals, and the general population to prioritize research, support services, and policy changes, advocacy becomes a catalyst for societal transformation in the face of Alzheimer's challenges.

## Grassroots Movements and Global Initiatives

This section underscores the transformative potential of grassroots movements and global initiatives in the realm of Alzheimer's. Grassroots advocacy, driven by communities, has the power to raise awareness, provide resources, and create networks of support. The discussion extends to global efforts, recognizing the interconnectedness of the challenges faced by societies worldwide.

The chapter highlights the significance of collaborative efforts involving governments, non-profit organizations, healthcare institutions, and individuals. By uniting in a shared commitment to combating Alzheimer's, societies can amplify their impact, foster innovation, and create a more supportive environment for those affected by the disease. The interconnected nature of global initiatives emphasizes the collective responsibility to address the multifaceted challenges posed by Alzheimer's on a global scale.

In conclusion, this chapter underscores the far-reaching implications of Alzheimer's on society, emphasizing the need for compassionate and informed responses. The social impact within families, workplaces, and economies necessitates a comprehensive and empathetic approach. Public awareness and advocacy are identified as potent tools for societal transformation, challenging stigmas and urging collaborative efforts to address the complex challenges posed by Alzheimer's on both a local and global level.

# Chapter 11: Future Perspectives

The landscape of Alzheimer's disease research and care is evolving, presenting a dynamic intersection of emerging technologies and a growing sense of hope for the future. This chapter delves into the transformative potential of cutting-edge technologies and the optimistic outlook that holds promise for individuals affected by Alzheimer's.

# Emerging Technologies

## Genomic Advancements and Personalized Therapies

In the realm of Alzheimer's research, genomic advancements stand at the forefront, offering a deeper understanding of the genetic underpinnings of the disease. Technologies such as CRISPR-Cas9 have ushered in an era of precision medicine, enabling scientists to manipulate specific genes associated with Alzheimer's. The potential for personalized therapies is explored, envisioning a future where treatments are tailored to an individual's unique genetic makeup. As genomic research progresses, the prospect of targeted interventions holds significant promise, offering a paradigm shift in the approach to Alzheimer's treatment.

## Artificial Intelligence in Diagnostics and Prediction

Artificial Intelligence (AI) emerges as a transformative force in the diagnosis and prediction of Alzheimer's. This subsection delves into how machine learning algorithms, fueled by vast datasets, including genetic information, biomarkers, and imaging results, analyze patterns to predict the risk of Alzheimer's. AI applications showcase their potential in revolutionizing early detection, providing more accurate and timely diagnoses. The exploration of AI's role in Alzheimer's care paints a picture of a future where predictive models may facilitate proactive interventions, offering a ray of hope for individuals at risk.

## Neurostimulation and Cognitive Enhancement

As technology advances, neurostimulation techniques emerge as potential interventions for Alzheimer's. Transcranial magnetic stimulation (TMS) and deep brain stimulation (DBS) are on the horizon, showing promise in modulating brain activity and potentially slowing cognitive decline. This section navigates the landscape of neurostimulation, exploring its potential role in enhancing cognitive functions and addressing the neurological changes associated with Alzheimer's. The discussion opens doors to innovative approaches that may reshape the traditional understanding of Alzheimer's care, offering hope for improved cognitive outcomes.

# Hope for the Future

## Targeting Disease-Modifying Therapies

Amidst the challenges presented by Alzheimer's, the pursuit of disease-modifying therapies provides a beacon of hope. This segment explores ongoing research efforts targeting the underlying mechanisms of the disease, such as the clearance of beta-amyloid plaques and the mitigation of neuroinflammation. While these therapies are in various stages of clinical trials, they hold the potential to alter the trajectory of Alzheimer's by addressing its root causes. The chapter acknowledges the persistence of challenges but underscores the optimism surrounding disease-modifying therapies as a transformative force in Alzheimer's research.

## Integrative Approaches and Holistic Care

Hope for the future extends beyond pharmaceutical breakthroughs, embracing integrative approaches and holistic care models. This part of the chapter explores the potential of combining medical interventions with lifestyle modifications, nutritional support, and psychological well-being strategies. The vision is of a future where individuals receive personalized and holistic care that transcends conventional treatment modalities. By recognizing the multifaceted nature of Alzheimer's, this approach aims to enhance the quality of life for affected individuals and provides hope for a more comprehensive and patient-centered care model.

## Empowering Communities and Reducing Stigma

The future of Alzheimer's is intrinsically tied to societal attitudes and support structures. This section emphasizes the importance of empowering communities to become more dementia-friendly and reducing the stigma associated with Alzheimer's. By fostering understanding and empathy, communities can play a crucial role in supporting individuals with Alzheimer's and their caregivers. The chapter envisions a future where societal awareness and advocacy efforts result in a more inclusive and compassionate environment, ultimately reducing the challenges faced by those affected by Alzheimer's.

In conclusion, the future perspectives on Alzheimer's disease are shaped by a dynamic interplay of emerging technologies, scientific advancements, and a collective vision for a more compassionate and supportive society. From genomic breakthroughs to the potential of artificial intelligence, the landscape of Alzheimer's research is evolving. Alongside scientific progress, hope for the future extends to holistic care approaches, disease-modifying therapies, and the empowerment of communities. As we navigate this complex terrain, the chapter encourages a collective commitment to shaping a future where the impact of Alzheimer's is minimized, and individuals affected by the disease find solace in a society that understands, supports, and strives for continued progress.

www.ingramcontent.com/pod-product-compliance
Lightning Source LLC
Chambersburg PA
CBHW071056290526
45795CB00004B/1516